FROM FEAR TO HOPE

Unveiling the Hidden Truths of Breast Cancer

Tony Ubah

Copyright

TABLE OF CONTENT

INTRODUCTION

In a world where information is at our fingertips, it's hard to imagine that there are still hidden truths lurking in the shadows.

Yet, when it comes to breast cancer, a disease that affects millions of women worldwide, there are still untold stories, unexplored avenues, and uncharted territories waiting to be discovered.

It is time to embark on a journey from fear to hope, as we unveil the hidden truths of breast cancer and empower ourselves with knowledge and understanding.

Breast cancer is a battle that many have fought, but few truly comprehend the depth of its impact. It is not just a disease that affects the physical body; it seeps into every facet of a person's life, leaving no stone unturned.

Beyond the realm of statistics and medical jargon lies a world of emotions, fears, and triumphs that remain unspoken. It is these hidden truths that we are here to uncover, for in understanding the whole picture, we can better support those who face this formidable foe.

This book is not a clinical guide filled with intimidating terminologies and impersonal facts.

No, it is a journey, a story woven with compassion, hope, and resilience. We will delve into the untold stories of breast cancer survivors, the unsung heroes who have braved the storm and emerged on the other side with newfound strength.

Their experiences will paint a vivid tapestry, illustrating the complex web of emotions and challenges that come with a diagnosis.

But this journey is not just for survivors; it is for anyone who has ever been touched by breast cancer, directly or indirectly. We will explore the perspectives of caregivers, families, and friends who play an indispensable role in the fight against this disease.

Their untold narratives will shed light on the importance of a strong support system and the power of love in the face of adversity.

Moreover, we will dig deep into the realm of scientific research, shedding light on the latest breakthroughs and discoveries that offer a glimmer of hope.

We will unravel the mysteries of genetic predispositions, environmental factors, and lifestyle choices, giving readers a comprehensive understanding of the factors that contribute to breast cancer development.

It is through this knowledge that we can empower ourselves and take proactive steps towards prevention and early detection.

But what sets this book apart from others is its commitment to unveiling the hidden truths. We will venture into the realm of taboo, exploring the sensitive topics that are often brushed under the rug.

From body image and sexuality to mental health and survivor's guilt, we will confront the challenges that breast cancer survivors face long after the battle is won.

By shining a light on these unspoken struggles, we hope to foster empathy, understanding, and support within our communities.

So, dear reader, are you ready to embark on this transformative journey from fear to hope? Are you willing to open your heart and mind to the hidden truths that lie within the world of breast cancer? Together, let us empower ourselves and those around us, igniting a flame of hope that will guide us towards a future where breast cancer is no longer a source of fear but a testament to the indomitable spirit of humanity.

Let the unveiling begin.

CHAPTER 1: The Silent Battle: Unmasking the Hidden Face of Breast Cancer

Dispelling Myths: Breaking Free from Misconceptions

In the realm of medical mysteries, breast cancer remains one of the most enigmatic and widely misunderstood diseases of our time. As shadows of ignorance continue to shroud this formidable opponent, it is crucial to shed light on the hidden face of breast cancer.

Join us on a captivating journey as we debunk misconceptions and unravel the truths that lie beneath the surface.

Myth #1: Breast Cancer Only Affects Women

Let's begin by dispelling a common myth: breast cancer is not a disease that discriminates based on gender. While it is true that women are disproportionately affected, breast cancer can also strike men.

Although rare, men possess breast tissue that can undergo malignant transformations. Shockingly, over 2,000 men are diagnosed with breast cancer each year in the United States alone. By unmasking this hidden face of breast cancer, we empower both women and men to recognize the importance of early detection and prevention.

Myth #2: Only Older Women Get Breast Cancer

Another myth we must shatter is the belief that breast cancer solely afflicts older women. While age is undeniably a risk factor, breast cancer can manifest at any stage of life.

In fact, a significant number of breast cancer cases occur in women under the age of 40. This revelation underscores the vital need for education and screening programs targeting younger demographics, ensuring that no one falls victim to this silent battle.

Myth #3: Breast Cancer is Always Detected through Lumps

Contrary to popular belief, breast cancer is not always heralded by palpable lumps. While lumps remain a common symptom, it is important to note that other signs may go unnoticed or unrecognized.

These can include changes in breast shape, nipple discharge, skin dimpling, or redness. Familiarizing ourselves with these lesser-known symptoms can be a game-changer in early detection, potentially saving lives.

The Shocking Reality: How Breast Cancer Affects Women and Men

Now that we have debunked some prevalent myths, let's delve into the staggering reality of breast cancer and how it impacts the lives of those who battle it.

Reality #1: Breast Cancer is a Global Epidemic

Breast cancer knows no borders; it is a global epidemic affecting millions worldwide. The World Health Organization estimates that over 2.3 million women were diagnosed with breast cancer in 2020 alone.

Furthermore, breast cancer remains the most common cancer among women globally, surpassing even lung cancer. These shocking statistics highlight the urgent need for international collaboration, increased research, and improved access to healthcare to combat this pervasive disease.

Reality #2: Breast Cancer Extends Beyond Physical Health

Breast cancer's impact stretches far beyond physical health, infiltrating the emotional, psychological, and social well-being of individuals and their families. The battle against breast cancer can lead to feelings of fear, anxiety, and depression.

Moreover, the financial burden associated with treatment and care can be overwhelming, exacerbating the emotional toll. By unmasking this hidden aspect of breast cancer, we open the dialogue for comprehensive support systems that address the multifaceted needs of patients and their loved ones.

Reality #3: Progress and Hope in the Face of Adversity

Amidst the challenging landscape of breast cancer, there is reason for hope. Advancements in medical research have paved the way for innovative treatments and early detection methods, improving survival rates and quality of life for many patients.

From targeted therapies to personalized medicine, the field of breast cancer research is at the forefront of groundbreaking discoveries. By fostering awareness and supporting ongoing research efforts, we can inspire the development of novel strategies and ultimately triumph over this hidden face of breast cancer, granting a brighter future for those affected.

The Silent Battle: Unmasking the Hidden Face of Breast Cancer invites you to embark on a captivating journey where knowledge becomes power. By dispelling myths and uncovering shocking realities, we break free from the chains of misconceptions, empowering ourselves and our communities to confront breast cancer head-on.

In the chapters to come, we will dive deeper into the intricate web of breast cancer, exploring risk factors, screening methods, treatment options, and the transformative power of support networks.

Through scientific facts, compelling narratives, and expert insights, we will unveil the hidden face of breast cancer, exposing its vulnerabilities and revealing the tools we possess to conquer it.

Imagine a world where breast cancer is no longer a silent battle, where misconceptions crumble in the face of truth, and where lives are saved through early detection and groundbreaking research.

This vision is within our reach, but it demands our engagement, our passion, and our hunger for knowledge.

Join us as we journey through the pages of this book, where the hidden face of breast cancer is unmasked, and the voices of survivors, researchers, and medical professionals come together to empower and inspire.

Together, let's illuminate the path toward a future where breast cancer is no longer a feared adversary but a conquered foe.

Prepare to be captivated by the scientific breakthroughs that defy conventional wisdom, the stories of resilience that defy statistics, and the triumphs that defy all odds.

Together, we will forge a new narrative, one that acknowledges the hidden face of breast cancer while emboldening us to rewrite its story.

So, arm yourself with knowledge, open your heart to empathy, and let curiosity guide you as we journey further into the depths of this silent battle. The hidden face of breast cancer will be revealed, and with it, the power to make a difference in the lives of those affected.

Are you ready to embark on this transformative journey? The pages ahead hold the key to understanding, compassion, and hope. Let us cast aside the veil of ignorance and shed light on the hidden face of breast cancer, for knowledge is our weapon, compassion our shield, and unity our strength.

Turn the page and let the revelations begin. The silent battle against breast cancer awaits, and together, we shall prevail.

CHAPTER 2: Unveiling the Enemy Within: Understanding the Causes and Risk Factors

Genetic Roulette: The Role of Hereditary Factors

Deep within the blueprint of our existence lies a hidden game of chance, a genetic roulette that shapes our very being. We may not realize it, but our genes hold the key to understanding many of the mysteries that surround us, including the enigmatic world of disease.

Welcome to the realm where nature and nurture collide, where the dice are cast long before we even take our first breath.

While we often think of genetics as a predetermined destiny, the truth is far more intricate. Our genetic makeup does play a pivotal role in determining our vulnerability to certain conditions, but it's not the sole dictator of our health.

Imagine a deck of cards, each representing a gene. Every hand we are dealt is unique, and it's the combination of these cards that ultimately shapes our genetic fate.

Genetic research has uncovered a labyrinth of gene variations, mutations, and interactions that can either confer protection or raise the odds of disease.

From the notorious BRCA genes associated with breast cancer to the apolipoprotein E (APOE) gene linked to Alzheimer's disease, these genetic markers serve as harbingers, warning us of potential dangers that lie ahead.

But here's the secret that many fail to realize: genes are not destiny. Our genetic makeup is like a roadmap, guiding us through life, but it's our lifestyle choices that determine the twists and turns we take.

Even if we carry genes associated with certain diseases, our environment and behavior can tip the scales in our favor.

The emerging field of epigenetics has shown us that we possess the power to influence our genetic expression through our everyday choices.

Environmental Factors: Unraveling the Silent Culprits

Picture a silent army of invaders infiltrating our bodies, wreaking havoc from within. They don't come armed with guns or swords, but with the invisible weapons of environmental factors.

These silent culprits surround us, lurking in the air we breathe, the water we drink, and the food we consume.
They are the hidden accomplices responsible for the rise of numerous diseases that plague modern society.

From the toxins in our environment to the stressors we encounter daily, our bodies are constantly under siege. Chemical pollutants, such as heavy metals, pesticides, and endocrine disruptors, infiltrate our systems and disrupt the delicate balance that keeps us healthy.

They stealthily interfere with our hormones, impair our immune defenses, and tip the scales towards disease.

But it's not just external factors that pose a threat. Our lifestyle choices also play a significant role in shaping our health outcomes.

Sedentary lifestyles, poor nutrition, and chronic stress are like allies of the enemy within, weakening our defenses and making us susceptible to a wide range of ailments.

Unveiling the truth about these environmental factors is crucial for our well-being. It empowers us to make informed decisions, to demand change, and to protect ourselves and future generations. We need to become vigilant warriors, armed with scientific facts, ready to face the silent culprits head-on.

Did you know that the air inside our homes can be more polluted than the air outside? Everyday items like cleaning products, furniture, and even the paint on our walls emit volatile organic compounds (VOCs) that can cause respiratory problems, allergies, and even cancer.

By understanding these hidden dangers, we can take steps to create a healthier indoor environment for ourselves and our loved ones.

And what about the food we consume? Industrial farming practices, pesticides, and food additives have turned our meals into a battleground.

Choosing organic produce and minimizing processed foods can shield us from harmful chemicals and additives, reducing the risk of chronic diseases like cancer, obesity, and diabetes.

Furthermore, stress, the invisible villain that infiltrates our lives, can wreak havoc on our health. Chronic stress triggers a cascade of physiological responses that compromise our immune system, increase inflammation, and raise the risk of cardiovascular disease, mental health disorders, and even premature aging.

By understanding the impact of stress on our bodies and adopting stress management techniques like meditation, exercise, and self-care, we can fortify our defenses and regain control over our well-being.

The enemy within is cunning and adaptable, but armed with knowledge, we can unveil their secrets and conquer their influence.
It's time to shed light on the silent culprits that operate in the shadows, to educate ourselves and others about the profound impact of our genes and our environment on our health.

In the chapters that follow, we will delve deeper into the intricate web of genetic and environmental factors, exploring the latest scientific discoveries and unveiling the connections between seemingly unrelated pieces of the puzzle.

We will uncover the remarkable interplay between nature and nurture, discovering how our genes interact with our environment, shaping our health outcomes.

But knowledge alone is not enough. It is the action we take that truly defines our journey. Armed with scientific facts and a burning desire for change, we have the power to rewrite our genetic narrative.

We can adopt healthier lifestyles, demand cleaner environments, and advocate for policies that prioritize the well-being of future generations.

Are you ready to join the fight against the enemy within? Are you hungry for knowledge that challenges the status quo and empowers you to take control of your health? Prepare yourself for an eye-opening journey, where we unravel the mysteries of our genes, expose the hidden dangers of our environment, and chart a path towards a healthier future.

In the next chapter, we will explore the intricate dance between genes and lifestyle choices, unveiling the power we possess to influence our genetic expression.

Get ready to embark on a quest that will challenge your preconceptions, expand your horizons, and ignite a passion for understanding the causes and risk factors that shape our lives.

Stay tuned as we unravel the enigma of our genetic roulette and expose the silent culprits lurking in our environment. Together, we can conquer the enemy within and pave the way for a brighter, healthier future.

CHAPTER 3

Unleash Your Genetic Symphony: The Hidden Dance of Genes and Lifestyle Choices

Have you ever wondered how much control you truly have over your genes? Buckle up, because we're about to embark on a mind-blowing journey into the mysterious world of genetic expression. Brace yourself for a revelation: your lifestyle choices possess a staggering power to shape the very essence of who you are!

We all know that our genes act as the blueprint for life, but what if I told you that they are not rigid, unyielding structures?

In fact, our genes possess a remarkable flexibility, responding and adapting to the rhythm of our daily choices. It's a captivating dance, where your lifestyle choices take the lead, and your genes gracefully follow suit.

You may be thinking, "But isn't my genetic destiny set in stone?" Not so fast! While we inherit certain genetic predispositions, it is our lifestyle choices that determine whether those genes manifest positively or negatively. It's like having a symphony within you, and you hold the conductor's baton.

Imagine this: your DNA, that intricate spiral of life, is studded with switches called "epigenetic markers."

These markers respond to environmental cues, signaling genes to turn on or off, dialing up or down their expression. Guess what? Your lifestyle choices can influence these epigenetic markers, orchestrating a symphony of health and vitality.

Let's dive into the scientific wonders that will leave you craving for more. Did you know that regular exercise can literally change the expression of your genes? Studies have shown that physical activity can enhance the production of proteins responsible for brain health, reducing the risk of cognitive decline.

So lace up those sneakers and let your genes groove to the rhythm of movement!

But the power doesn't stop there. Your nutritional choices have the ability to harmonize your genes like never before. Certain foods, like colorful fruits and vegetables, burst with antioxidants that protect your DNA from damage, while others, like omega-3 fatty acids, can fine-tune gene expression for optimal heart health.

It's time to embrace the art of mindful eating and savor the symphony of flavors that nourish your genes.

And hold your breath, because stress management is the conductor's baton that can truly transform your genetic symphony.

Chronic stress, like an off-key note, can wreak havoc on your gene expression, leading to a host of health issues. But fear not! Mindfulness practices, meditation, and relaxation techniques can harmonize those stress-induced genetic discordances, allowing your genes to sing in perfect harmony.

So, dear reader, are you hungry for more? The intricate dance between genes and lifestyle choices is an awe-inspiring tale of empowerment.

It's a story that challenges the notion of genetic determinism, reminding us that we possess the incredible ability to mold our genetic destiny through everyday decisions.

Unlock the secrets within you and discover the power you hold to influence your genetic expression. Step onto the stage of your life and let your genes waltz to the beat of a healthier, happier you. Embrace the beauty of this hidden dance and let it become the soundtrack of your vibrant existence.

Are you ready to embark on this thrilling adventure? Stay tuned for the next chapter, Let the dance begin!

CHAPTER 4: The Road Less Traveled: Navigating Diagnosis and Treatment

The Dreaded Diagnosis: Facing the Moment of Truth

In the realm of healthcare, few words strike fear into the hearts of individuals more than "diagnosis." It's the moment of truth, the instant when our lives can change forever.

The emotions that accompany a diagnosis are complex, ranging from disbelief to anxiety, and from fear to determination. But amidst this sea of emotions, it's important to arm ourselves with knowledge and face the situation head-on.

What many people don't realize is that a diagnosis is not a final verdict, but rather a starting point on a challenging journey. Medical advancements have propelled us far beyond the days when a diagnosis meant a bleak prognosis.

Today, precision medicine, genomics, and cutting-edge technologies are revolutionizing the way we understand and treat diseases.

As daunting as it may seem, taking an active role in understanding your diagnosis is crucial. Seeking a second opinion can provide invaluable insights, as different doctors may have unique perspectives and treatment approaches.

Remember, knowledge is power, and the more you understand about your condition, the better equipped you are to make informed decisions.

Treatment Options: Beyond Surgery, Chemotherapy, and Radiation

When we think of cancer treatment, the usual suspects come to mind: surgery, chemotherapy, and radiation. But did you know that these traditional treatments represent just the tip of the iceberg? The field of oncology has been steadily advancing, and a vast array of innovative and tailored treatment options now exist.

One such breakthrough is immunotherapy, a cutting-edge approach that harnesses the power of our own immune system to fight cancer. By stimulating and enhancing the body's natural defenses, immunotherapy has shown remarkable success in treating various cancers, even those that were once considered untreatable.

It's a shining beacon of hope for patients who have exhausted conventional treatment options.

Another promising avenue lies in targeted therapies, which specifically attack cancer cells while sparing healthy ones. These therapies capitalize on the unique genetic makeup of tumors, homing in on specific molecular abnormalities.

By blocking the signals that fuel cancer growth, targeted therapies can effectively halt the disease's progression, often with fewer side effects than traditional treatments.

The world of oncology is also embracing precision medicine, an approach that takes into account individual variations in genes, environment, and lifestyle.

Through advanced genomic analysis, doctors can now tailor treatments to the specific characteristics of a patient's tumor. This personalized approach holds tremendous potential, ensuring that each patient receives the most effective treatment with the fewest adverse effects.

But it's not just cancer that benefits from groundbreaking treatments. In the realm of neurology, for example, deep brain stimulation has emerged as a remarkable tool for managing conditions such as Parkinson's disease and essential tremor.

By implanting electrodes deep within the brain and providing controlled electrical stimulation, this technique can alleviate symptoms and improve patients' quality of life.

Beyond traditional medicine, complementary therapies and integrative approaches are gaining recognition for their potential to support conventional treatments.

Practices like acupuncture, meditation, and yoga have been shown to alleviate treatment-related side effects, reduce stress, and improve overall well-being. Integrating these practices into a comprehensive care plan can foster a holistic healing environment for patients.

As we navigate the road less traveled in diagnosis and treatment, it's essential to remember that hope springs eternal. The landscape of healthcare is rapidly evolving, with breakthroughs occurring every day.

The dreaded diagnosis may mark the beginning of a challenging journey, but

armed with knowledge and empowered by innovative treatment options,
we can navigate this path with newfound confidence.

So, when faced with a diagnosis, remember to seek knowledge, consult multiple experts, and explore beyond the conventional.

Embrace the power of precision medicine, targeted therapies, and immunotherapy. Consider complementary and integrative approaches that can enhance your well-being.

Embrace the potential of breakthrough technologies like deep brain stimulation. Open your mind to the possibilities that lie beyond the familiar realms of surgery, chemotherapy, and radiation.

It's important to understand that no two journeys are the same. Each person's diagnosis and treatment path are unique, and what works for one may not work for another. That's why it's crucial to have open and honest conversations with your healthcare team, discussing all available options and weighing the risks and benefits.

Remember, scientific advancements are driven by tireless researchers and dedicated healthcare professionals who are constantly pushing the boundaries of what is possible.

They are unraveling the mysteries of diseases and uncovering new treatment avenues. By staying informed and engaged, you become an active participant in your own healing journey.

Additionally, don't underestimate the power of support systems. Seek out patient advocacy groups, connect with others who have gone through similar experiences, and surround yourself with loved ones who can provide the emotional support you need.

Together, you can find strength, share knowledge, and navigate the challenges that lie ahead.It's also essential to address the emotional and psychological aspects of a diagnosis. Seeking counseling or therapy can help you cope with the rollercoaster of emotions that often accompany a life-altering diagnosis.

Emotional well-being is an integral part of your overall health, and addressing it can enhance your resilience and ability to face the road ahead. In the face of a diagnosis, it's natural to feel overwhelmed and uncertain. But remember, there is hope. Breakthroughs in diagnosis and treatment are happening every day.

The road less traveled may be filled with twists and turns, but it also holds the promise of new discoveries and possibilities. So, let's embark on this journey together, armed with knowledge, empowered by science, and fueled by hope.

Embrace the road less traveled, for it is on this path that we may find the answers we seek, the treatments we need, and the healing we deserve.As we venture forth, let curiosity guide us, let determination fuel us, and let resilience sustain us.

Together, we can navigate the uncharted territories of diagnosis and treatment, emerging stronger, wiser, and filled with a renewed appreciation for the resilience of the human spirit.So, take a deep breath, gather your strength, and step onto the road less traveled. Your journey awaits, and the possibilities are endless.

Let's embark on this adventure with hope in our hearts and a determination to carve a path towards healing and a brighter future.

As you turn the page to the next chapter, remember that you are not alone. Countless others have traveled this road before you, and many more will follow. Together, we can rewrite the narrative of diagnosis and treatment, uncovering new possibilities, and paving the way for a world where diseases are conquered, and lives are transformed.

The road less traveled beckons, and it's time to embark on this extraordinary journey of healing and discovery.

Let's walk this path together, as we navigate the uncharted territories of diagnosis and treatment, hand in hand, towards a future filled with hope and possibility.

CHAPTER 5 Empowered Warriors: Stories of Triumph and Resilience

Strength in Vulnerability: Inspirational Tales of Survivors

In a world that often values invulnerability and steadfastness, there lies an uncharted territory of strength — vulnerability. Behind the seemingly impenetrable facades of everyday warriors, there exists an untold power, hidden within the depths of their resilience.

These are the untold stories of triumph, showcasing the indomitable human spirit that rises from the depths of vulnerability.

Meet Sarah, a survivor of a near-fatal accident that left her paralyzed from the waist down. Many would assume that such a life-altering event would shatter her spirit, leaving her broken and defeated.

However, Sarah's story is one of resilience and the immense power found within vulnerability. Through embracing her new reality, Sarah tapped into her innate strength, overcoming physical limitations and proving that disability does not define her.

Scientifically, this strength lies in the human brain's remarkable ability to adapt and rewire itself, known as neuroplasticity.

When faced with adversity, the brain rewires its neural connections, allowing individuals like Sarah to find new pathways and regain control over their lives. Sarah's journey serves as a powerful testament to the fact that strength in vulnerability is not only possible but also life-changing.

Another remarkable story of triumph is that of Michael, who battled against a long-standing addiction. Addiction is often stigmatized and misunderstood, with many failing to comprehend the immense strength required to overcome it.

Michael's journey showcases the inherent power found within vulnerability and the unwavering resilience that can be harnessed to overcome even the most challenging obstacles.

Behind the scenes, our brain's reward system plays a vital role in addiction and recovery. Drugs hijack this system, creating a vicious cycle that can seem impossible to break.

However, recent scientific studies have revealed that social support and human connection are key factors in successful addiction recovery.

Michael's story is a testament to the unbreakable bonds formed within support networks, as he leaned on loved ones, therapy, and community to triumph over his addiction and rediscover his true self.

Unbreakable Bonds: The Support Network that Changes Lives

In the realm of triumph and resilience, one cannot underestimate the power of human connection. Behind the scenes of every victorious battle lies an army of unwavering support, forming unbreakable bonds that change lives forever.

These stories illuminate the true essence of humanity and the transformative power of love, compassion, and understanding.

Meet Emma, a survivor of domestic violence, who found solace and strength in the support network that rallied around her. Behind closed doors, Emma's life was a harrowing tale of abuse and fear.

Yet, her journey toward healing and empowerment began when she mustered the courage to confide in a trusted friend. It was through this first act of vulnerability that she unlocked the immense power of connection.

With the support of her friends, family, and community organizations, Emma emerged as a beacon of resilience and a testament to the life-altering impact of support networks.

Scientifically, the power of social connection is backed by numerous studies that highlight its profound impact on mental and physical well-being. From reducing stress hormones to boosting the immune system, human connection is a fundamental human need that can make all the difference in one's journey toward triumph.

These stories of empowered warriors are but a glimpse into the untold narratives of strength in vulnerability and the unbreakable bonds forged in support networks. Beyond the facade of invulnerability, there lies a wealth of stories waiting to be heard, each one brimming with resilience, triumph, and the remarkable power of human connection.

As we delve further into these tales of triumph, we'll discover the extraordinary potential that lies within us all. From the depths of despair to the pinnacle of victory, these stories inspire us to embrace our vulnerabilities and tap into the reservoirs of strength that reside within.

Take the story of David, a survivor of a traumatic brain injury. When an accident left him with cognitive impairments and limited mobility, David faced a daunting journey to reclaim his life.

Yet, it was through his vulnerability and the support of his loved ones that he found the resilience to adapt and thrive.

Scientifically, the brain's ability to heal and adapt, known as neuroplasticity, played a pivotal role in David's recovery. Through intensive therapy, rehabilitation, and unwavering support, David rewired his neural pathways, defying the odds and rewriting his own narrative.

But it is not just the individuals themselves who embody triumph; it is also the bonds formed within their support networks that catalyze their transformation.

These networks become lifelines, providing strength, empathy, and encouragement when it is needed most. From friends who lend a listening ear to professionals who offer guidance, the collective power of support networks is immeasurable.

Consider the story of Maria, a single mother battling cancer. Throughout her grueling treatment, Maria found solace and strength in a community of survivors and caregivers who understood her struggles firsthand.

The shared experiences, encouragement, and collective wisdom within this support network became a lifeline for Maria, empowering her to persevere and find hope even in the darkest of times.

Scientific studies have shown that social support not only improves emotional well-being but also positively impacts physical health outcomes, enhancing the body's ability to heal and recover.

These stories of triumph and resilience remind us that vulnerability is not synonymous with weakness. Instead, it is a testament to the courage and inner strength required to face adversity head-on. It is a reminder that within our vulnerabilities lie the seeds of growth, transformation, and unimaginable triumph.

As we navigate our own journeys, these stories compel us to reflect on our own vulnerabilities and the support networks that surround us. They urge us to embrace our own stories of resilience and seek the support we need to overcome obstacles.

Whether it be reaching out to a trusted friend, seeking professional help, or joining a community of like-minded individuals, we can tap into the wellspring of strength that lies within the power of connection.

In this chapter, we have embarked on a journey through the uncharted territories of triumph and resilience. We have witnessed the incredible power of vulnerability, the astounding adaptability of the human brain, and the transformative strength of support networks.

These stories of empowered warriors inspire us to rewrite our own narratives, to embrace our vulnerabilities, and to forge unbreakable bonds that carry us through the storms of life.

As we turn the pages and delve deeper into the lives of these remarkable individuals, we will uncover the secrets of their triumphs and witness the extraordinary resilience that resides within us all. These stories are not just tales of inspiration; they are powerful reminders that within every challenge lies the potential for growth, healing, and triumph.

So, let us embark on this journey together, and may these stories of empowered warriors ignite a fire within us all to embrace our vulnerabilities, seek support, and become the heroes of our own stories.

For in the face of adversity, there is triumph, and in the embrace of vulnerability, there is strength beyond measure.

CHAPTER 6 : Innovations in the Battle: Revolutionary Breakthroughs in Breast Cancer Research

Unlocking the Mysteries: The Promise of Genomic Medicine

In a world where technological advancements are rewriting the rules of medicine, the quest to conquer breast cancer has reached an unprecedented stage.

While this formidable disease has plagued women for centuries, a glimmer of hope has emerged from the depths of scientific exploration.

Prepare to be astonished as we unveil the hidden realm of genomic medicine, a cutting-edge field that is revolutionizing our understanding of breast cancer.

For years, researchers tirelessly hunted for answers, seeking to unravel the intricate web of genetic mutations that fuel the growth of cancer cells. The key to victory lay hidden within the blueprint of our very being—the human genome.

With remarkable precision, scientists have deciphered the secrets embedded within our

DNA, unmasking the intricate dance between genes and cancer development.

Every individual's genetic makeup contains vital clues that not only unlock the mysteries of breast cancer but also hold the key to highly personalized treatments.

But what exactly does this mean for patients battling breast cancer? It means that no longer are we confined to a one-size-fits-all approach.

Genomic medicine empowers doctors to delve into the depths of a patient's genetic profile, enabling them to tailor treatments to their unique biological makeup. By identifying specific genetic abnormalities within tumors, physicians can select targeted therapies that attack cancer cells with unrivaled precision.

This groundbreaking approach not only improves the effectiveness of treatment but also minimizes side effects, ensuring a better quality of life for patients.

From Lab to Life: Groundbreaking Therapies and Immunotherapies

Imagine a world where the immune system becomes an unstoppable force, a vigilant guardian against the insidious nature of breast cancer. This dream is fast becoming a reality with the advent of groundbreaking therapies and immunotherapies that harness the body's own defenses to combat this devastating disease.

Traditionally, cancer treatments have relied on chemotherapy, radiation, and surgery. While effective, these methods often come with debilitating side effects, leaving patients physically and emotionally drained. Enter immunotherapy, a game-changing approach that supercharges the immune system, enabling it to recognize and annihilate cancer cells with remarkable precision.

One such innovation that has taken the world by storm is immune checkpoint inhibitors. These groundbreaking drugs unleash the full potential of the immune system by disabling the brakes that cancer cells exploit to evade detection.

By liberating the immune system from its restraints, these inhibitors empower it to launch an all-out assault on cancer cells, leading to remarkable breakthroughs in breast cancer treatment.

Furthermore, scientists have pioneered the use of CAR-T cell therapy, an extraordinary technique that involves engineering a patient's own immune cells to specifically target cancer cells.

These modified cells are equipped with receptors that seek out and destroy cancerous invaders, leaving healthy tissue unharmed. The results are staggering, with patients experiencing dramatic responses and even achieving complete remission in some cases.

But the innovations do not stop there. Picture a world where we can predict a patient's response to treatment before it even begins. Enter liquid biopsies, a non-invasive technique that analyzes circulating tumor DNA (ctDNA) in a patient's blood.

This groundbreaking technology provides a wealth of information, allowing physicians to monitor treatment response in real-time and make timely adjustments for optimal outcomes.

Furthermore, it holds the potential to detect the recurrence of cancer at its earliest stages, opening doors to earlier intervention and greater chances of long-term survival.

As we venture further into the realm of breast cancer research, the possibilities seem endless. From targeted therapies based on genomic profiles to immune system revolutions and innovative detection methods, we are witnessing a revolution in the fight against breast cancer.

The age-old enemy is no longer invincible; it is now confronted by an arsenal of precision weapons that promise to tip the scales in favor of patients worldwide.

But this battle is not fought by scientists alone; it requires the collective efforts of healthcare providers, policymakers, and society as a whole.

Imagine a world where breast cancer is not just treated, but prevented altogether. This tantalizing vision may soon become a reality with groundbreaking advancements in cancer prevention.

Researchers are unraveling the complex interplay between genetics, lifestyle factors, and environmental exposures, paving the way for personalized risk assessment and targeted interventions.

By identifying individuals with a higher susceptibility to breast cancer, preventive measures such as lifestyle modifications, chemoprevention, and prophylactic surgeries can be employed to nip this silent killer in the bud.

Moreover, the power of collaboration and data sharing cannot be underestimated. As researchers across the globe pool their knowledge and resources, the pace of progress accelerates exponentially.

This collaborative spirit has given rise to initiatives such as The Cancer Genome Atlas (TCGA), a monumental effort that has mapped the genetic landscape of breast cancer, uncovering crucial insights into its biology and potential vulnerabilities.

But the fight against breast cancer goes beyond the realm of science and medicine. It is a battle that requires awareness, education, and support.

By empowering individuals with knowledge about risk factors, early detection methods, and treatment options, we equip them to become active participants in their own health journeys.

Furthermore, fostering a supportive environment for survivors and their families is paramount, as it nurtures hope, resilience, and the belief that victory is within reach.

As we turn the pages of history, we witness the unfolding of a new chapter in the battle against breast cancer. It is a chapter characterized by groundbreaking innovations, awe-inspiring scientific discoveries, and a relentless pursuit of a world free from the grip of this formidable disease.

Genomic medicine and targeted therapies hold the promise of personalized treatments, immunotherapies unleash the power of the immune system, and novel detection methods offer hope for early intervention.

The stage is set for a revolution, one where breast cancer bows before the might of human ingenuity and determination.

But this chapter is not yet complete. It is a call to action for researchers to continue their tireless pursuit of knowledge, for healthcare providers to embrace these cutting-edge technologies, and for society to rally behind the cause.

It is a reminder that each and every one of us has a role to play in this battle, whether it is through raising awareness, supporting research initiatives, or advocating for better access to care.So let us embark on this journey together, armed with knowledge and unwavering determination. Let us push the boundaries of what is possible and defy the limitations imposed by breast cancer.

The road ahead may be challenging, but the rewards are immeasurable. It is a road that leads to a future where breast cancer is no longer a devastating diagnosis but a conquerable foe. With every breakthrough, every innovation, and every life saved, we move closer to that triumphant moment when breast cancer is relegated to the annals of medical history.

CHAPTER 7: Healing Beyond the Physical: Nurturing the Mind, Body, and Soul

Mindfulness and Meditation: Harnessing the Power of Inner Peace

In our fast-paced and demanding world, it's easy to get caught up in the chaos of everyday life. We often neglect the most important aspect of our being: our mind.

But what if I told you that unlocking the power of your mind could lead to profound healing and transformation? Welcome to the world of mindfulness and meditation, where inner peace becomes the key to unlocking your full potential.

Mindfulness is the practice of paying attention to the present moment, cultivating awareness of your thoughts, feelings, and bodily sensations without judgment. It has been embraced by ancient traditions for centuries, and now modern science is catching up, revealing its incredible benefits.

Numerous studies have shown that mindfulness reduces stress, anxiety, and depression, while improving focus, memory, and overall well-being.

But what about the brain? How does mindfulness affect our most vital organ? Neuroscientists have discovered that regular meditation actually changes the structure and function of the brain.

It increases the density of gray matter in regions associated with emotional regulation, empathy, and self-awareness. It also strengthens the prefrontal cortex, the area responsible for decision-making, attention, and problem-solving.

Moreover, meditation has a profound impact on our physical health. It reduces inflammation in the body, lowers blood pressure, and enhances the immune system.

One study even found that meditation can influence the expression of genes related to stress and inflammation, effectively turning off harmful genes and activating beneficial ones.

But the benefits of mindfulness and meditation extend far beyond the individual. When we cultivate inner peace and emotional balance, we become more compassionate and empathetic towards others.

Research shows that mindfulness practice increases feelings of connectedness and social engagement, leading to stronger relationships and a greater sense of belonging.

Embracing Life After Cancer: Reclaiming Joy and Wellness

Receiving a cancer diagnosis is a life-altering event. It challenges not only the physical body but also the very fabric of our existence.

The journey through cancer treatment is undoubtedly difficult, but what many don't realize is that life after cancer can be just as challenging, if not more so. Yet, within this struggle lies an opportunity for immense growth and profound joy.

Reclaiming joy and wellness after cancer begins with understanding that healing is a holistic process. It involves nurturing the mind, body, and soul.

Scientific research has shown that individuals who engage in activities such as exercise, healthy eating, and mind-body practices have a higher quality of life and better overall well-being after cancer treatment.

Exercise, for instance, has been found to not only improve physical strength and stamina but also reduce fatigue, anxiety, and depression. It boosts the production of endorphins, the body's natural feel-good chemicals, promoting a sense of happiness and well-being.

Additionally, regular exercise has been linked to a lower risk of cancer recurrence and improved long-term survival rates.

When it comes to nutrition, adopting a balanced and nourishing diet can have a profound impact on post-cancer recovery.

Research suggests that a diet rich in fruits, vegetables, whole grains, and lean proteins can reduce the risk of cancer recurrence and enhance overall health. Furthermore, certain foods, such as turmeric, green tea, and cruciferous vegetables, possess powerful anti-cancer properties, providing an extra layer of protection.

However, true healing after cancer goes beyond the physical realm. It involves nurturing the soul and finding meaning in the experience.

Many cancer survivors report a renewed sense of purpose and a deeper appreciation for life after facing their mortality.

Engaging in activities that bring joy and fulfillment, such as spending time in nature, pursuing creative outlets, or connecting with loved ones, can foster a profound sense of well-being and ignite a spark of resilience within.

It's important to acknowledge that the emotional and psychological impact of cancer can be long-lasting. Many survivors experience anxiety, depression, and post-traumatic stress disorder (PTSD) following their treatment.

This is where therapy and support groups play a crucial role in the healing journey.

Cognitive-behavioral therapy (CBT) and other evidence-based approaches can help individuals process their emotions, develop coping strategies, and cultivate a positive mindset.

In recent years, complementary therapies such as acupuncture, yoga, and massage have gained recognition for their ability to support cancer survivors in their quest for wellness.

Acupuncture, for example, has been shown to alleviate treatment-related symptoms such as pain, nausea, and fatigue. It also promotes relaxation and balances the body's energy system, enhancing overall well-being.

Yoga, on the other hand, combines physical movement, breathwork, and mindfulness to create a holistic practice that nurtures both the body and mind.

Numerous studies have demonstrated the benefits of yoga for cancer survivors, including improved sleep, reduced stress, and increased flexibility and strength. Yoga also provides a safe space for survivors to reconnect with their bodies and cultivate self-compassion.

Massage therapy, known for its ability to relax muscles and reduce tension, offers cancer survivors a much-needed respite from the physical and emotional toll of their journey. It can alleviate pain, improve sleep quality, and enhance the immune system.

Additionally, the nurturing touch of a skilled massage therapist can provide comfort and emotional support, helping survivors feel seen and cared for.

As the scientific understanding of the mind-body-soul connection deepens, an integrative approach to healing is emerging. It recognizes that true wellness encompasses all aspects of our being and encourages individuals to explore a wide range of modalities.

From music therapy to art therapy, from journaling to spiritual practices, there are countless paths to healing waiting to be discovered.

Reclaiming joy and wellness after cancer is a deeply personal journey. It requires courage, resilience, and a willingness to embrace life's uncertainties. It's about finding balance and creating a life that aligns with your values and passions. It's about celebrating every moment, big or small, and cherishing the gift of each new day.

So, if you find yourself on the path of post-cancer recovery, remember that you are not alone. Reach out to support networks, explore integrative therapies, and above all, be gentle with yourself.

Embrace the journey of healing beyond the physical, and you'll discover a wellspring of resilience, joy, and strength within you that you never knew existed.

In the next chapter, we will explore the Advocacy for Change: Transforming the Breast Cancer Landscape
- Raising Awareness: Fighting Stigma and Taboos
- The Future of Breast Cancer: A Call to Action
 and its profound impact on our well-being. Prepare to embark on this journey that will elevate your life to new heights.

CHAPTER 8: Advocacy for Change: Transforming the Breast Cancer Landscape

Raising Awareness: Fighting Stigma and Taboos

Breast cancer, a disease that affects millions of women worldwide, continues to be shrouded in stigma and taboos. It's time to break free from the chains of silence and raise awareness about this prevalent illness that touches the lives of so many.

Let's delve into the untold truths and scientific facts that people often overlook, shedding light on the real impact of breast cancer and the urgent need for change.

Did you know that breast cancer is not just a disease that affects women? While it's true that women are the most commonly affected, men can also develop breast cancer, albeit at a lower rate. By dismissing this fact, we perpetuate the misconception that breast cancer is solely a female problem.

Advocacy for change demands that we recognize the inclusivity of breast cancer and provide support to all those affected, irrespective of gender.

Furthermore, it's crucial to debunk the myths surrounding breast cancer, as misinformation can be detrimental to early detection and treatment. One prevalent myth is that only older women are at risk.

The truth is that breast cancer can strike at any age, including younger women. By raising awareness among all age groups, we empower women to be proactive about their breast health and seek timely screenings and check-ups.

Let's also challenge the notion that breast cancer is always accompanied by a noticeable lump.

While lumps are a common symptom, other signs, such as changes in breast size or shape, skin dimpling, nipple discharge, or persistent pain, should not be ignored.

Understanding the various manifestations of breast cancer enables individuals to be vigilant and seek medical attention promptly, potentially saving lives.

As we look ahead to the future of breast cancer, it's clear that a call to action is needed. Despite significant advancements in research and treatment, breast cancer remains a formidable adversary.

Here are some scientific facts that highlight the urgency for change and innovation:

1. **Precision Medicine**: Every breast cancer is unique, and tailoring treatments to individual patients' specific genetic and molecular profiles holds tremendous promise.

Through precision medicine, scientists aim to develop targeted therapies that maximize efficacy while minimizing side effects. This approach brings hope for improved treatment outcomes and better quality of life for breast cancer patients.

2. **Liquid Biopsies**: Traditional biopsies involve invasive procedures, causing discomfort and anxiety.

However, emerging liquid biopsy techniques offer a less invasive alternative. By analyzing circulating tumor DNA or tumor cells present in the blood, liquid biopsies provide valuable insights into a patient's cancer status, aiding in early detection, monitoring treatment response, and identifying potential resistance mechanisms.

3. **Immunotherapy**: Harnessing the power of the immune system to fight cancer has revolutionized cancer treatment. While immunotherapy has shown remarkable success in various cancers, its potential in breast cancer is yet to be fully realized. Ongoing research aims to uncover new

immunotherapeutic targets specific to breast cancer, paving the way for innovative treatment strategies.

4. **Prevention and Risk Reduction**: Prevention is always better than cure, and breast cancer is no exception. Lifestyle modifications, including maintaining a healthy weight, regular physical activity, limiting alcohol consumption, and avoiding tobacco, can significantly reduce the risk of breast cancer.

By emphasizing prevention and risk reduction strategies, we can empower individuals to take control of their breast health.

5. **Global Collaboration**: Breast cancer knows no borders. International collaboration among researchers, healthcare professionals, and policymakers is essential for driving progress in breast cancer research, prevention, and treatment. By sharing knowledge, resources, and expertise, we can accelerate breakthroughs and create a global impact in the fight against breast cancer.

As we conclude this chapter, it's clear that advocacy for change is the key to transforming the breast cancer landscape. We must strive to create a society that is knowledgeable, empathetic, and proactive in addressing this disease.

By raising awareness, challenging stigmas, and embracing scientific advancements, we can make a real difference in the lives of those affected by breast cancer.

Education and awareness campaigns are powerful tools in dismantling the stigma surrounding breast cancer. We need to engage communities, schools, workplaces, and the media to promote open conversations about breast health, encouraging regular screenings and self-examinations.

By dispelling myths and addressing misconceptions, we empower individuals to make informed decisions about their health and seek timely medical attention.

Additionally, it's crucial to provide a supportive environment for breast cancer patients and survivors. Breast cancer can be physically, emotionally, and socially challenging, and survivors often face discrimination, body image issues, and mental health struggles.

By fostering a culture of compassion and understanding, we can create a safe space where individuals can share their experiences, seek support, and access resources that enhance their well-being.

In parallel with raising awareness, scientific advancements and research must continue to drive progress in breast cancer prevention, detection, and treatment.

This requires sustained investment in research programs, clinical trials, and cutting-edge technologies.

Governments, organizations, and individuals alike must rally together to provide the necessary resources and funding to fuel these endeavors.

Advancements such as precision medicine, liquid biopsies, immunotherapy, and risk reduction strategies offer hope for a future where breast cancer becomes a more manageable and curable disease.

However, turning these scientific breakthroughs into accessible and affordable treatments requires collaboration between researchers, pharmaceutical companies, and regulatory bodies.

By streamlining the process of bringing innovations from the lab to the clinic, we can ensure that patients receive the best care possible.

Furthermore, global collaboration is paramount in the fight against breast cancer. The sharing of knowledge, data, and expertise across borders accelerates progress and prevents redundant efforts.

International organizations and research networks play a vital role in facilitating collaboration and fostering a sense of unity among scientists, healthcare professionals, and policymakers. By working together, we can achieve greater impact and reach underserved populations with limited access to healthcare.

In conclusion, transforming the breast cancer landscape requires a multi-faceted approach encompassing education, advocacy, scientific research, and global collaboration.

By raising awareness, fighting stigma and taboos, embracing scientific advancements, and fostering global cooperation, we can create a future where breast cancer is detected early, treated effectively, and ultimately prevented.

Let us stand together in this fight, armed with knowledge, compassion, and a shared determination to make a positive change. The time for action is now, and the future of breast cancer depends on our unwavering commitment to advocacy for change.

CONCLUSION

In a world where fear often pervades discussions surrounding breast cancer, it is time to unveil the hidden truths and transform that fear into hope.

"From Fear to Hope" takes you on an extraordinary journey, diving deep into the intricacies of breast cancer, shedding light on the secrets that have been overlooked for far too long.

This book has aimed to empower lives and inspire change, inviting readers to challenge their perceptions and embrace a new understanding of this complex disease.

Throughout these pages, we have embarked on an enlightening expedition, unearthing scientific facts that have the power to revolutionize our approach to breast cancer.

From the role of genetics to the impact of environmental factors, we have explored the multifaceted nature of this disease, breaking free from misconceptions and embracing a wealth of knowledge that has the potential to save lives.

One of the astonishing revelations uncovered in this journey is the importance of early detection. Armed with the knowledge that regular mammograms can detect breast cancer at its earliest stages, readers now have the tools to take control of their own health.

Gone are the days of fear and uncertainty; we are now equipped with the power of prevention, armed with the understanding that early intervention can lead to increased chances of survival and successful treatment.

Furthermore, we have delved into the realm of personalized medicine, where groundbreaking advancements are transforming the landscape of breast cancer treatment.

By harnessing the power of genomic sequencing, researchers and physicians can tailor treatments to individual patients, ensuring greater efficacy and reducing unnecessary side effects.

This personalized approach brings hope to patients, providing them with the reassurance that their journey through breast cancer will be met with the most effective and targeted interventions.

In our exploration, we have shattered the stigma that surrounds breast cancer. No longer should it be whispered behind closed doors; it is time to bring this disease out into the open, encouraging open dialogue and fostering a sense of community.

By embracing hope, we can create a support network that empowers individuals and offers solace to those affected.

From survivor stories that inspire courage to the tireless efforts of researchers and healthcare professionals, this book celebrates the triumph of the human spirit and the determination to conquer breast cancer.

However, our journey does not end here. As we conclude this captivating narrative, it is important to recognize that the fight against breast cancer is far from over. Each page turned and each truth uncovered should serve as a call to action.

We must continue to invest in research, advocate for comprehensive healthcare, and promote awareness campaigns that reach every corner of the globe.

By doing so, we can eradicate the hidden truths that have plagued our society for too long.

Dear reader, as you close the final chapter of "From Fear to Hope," may you carry with you a newfound understanding, an unwavering hope, and an insatiable hunger for more knowledge.

Let the hidden truths revealed in these pages ignite a fire within you, propelling you to be a champion of change. Together, we can transform fear into hope, empower lives, and inspire a future free from the grips of breast cancer. The journey continues, and it is our collective responsibility to forge a path towards a brighter, healthier tomorrow.